Atkins Diet

Cookbook

Soups & Salads

44 Easy and Delicious Recipes to Help You Lose Weight and Improve Your Health

Maggie Vega

Table of Contents

4

Introduction

What is the Atkins Diet?

It is basically a low-carbs diet termed as Atkins Diet after the name of the physician Dr. Robert C. Atkins who promoted it in the year 1972. He also wrote a book in the same year to guide people with the diet.

The Atkins diet allows minimum intake of the carbohydrates so that body's metabolism boosts which helps in the burning of body's fat to produce energy and body undergo a process of ketosis. Ketosis process starts with the lower insulin levels in the body causing the consumption and burning of the fats to generate ketone bodies. On contrary, consumption of higher carbohydrates increases blood sugar levels thus accumulation of the fats occurs.

Atkins diet promotes simple eating habits which reduces the appetite. Atkins diet foods are rich in fats and proteins thus longer duration of digestion is required which lowers the raise of hunger.

Formerly, the Atkins diet was considered unhealthy because of the high saturated fat intake but recent research has proved it harmless. In fact the high consumption of high fat diet like Atkins diet has shown tremendous health improvements like lowering the blood sugar levels, cholesterol levels, triglycerides and makes you tidy up to look smarter and fresh. The main reason that is most appealing to use this diet is that it is helpful in lowering done your appetite which vanishes with a little intake of calories.

The Atkins Diet Plan

The Atkins diet is usually split up into 4 different phases with each phase with different food items:

Induction phase (phase 1): This phase of the diet is quite tough as one has to intake less than 20 grams of carbs each day for 2 weeks. High proteins and fats are encouraged to eat with leaf green vegetables that contain low carbohydrates. These healthy weeks will start your weight loss.

Balancing Phase (phase 2): In this phase, try to create a equilibrium in your diet by slowly adding low-carb vegetables, more nuts, and a little amount of fruit back in your food.

1. Fine-Tuning Phase (phase 3): Seeing yourself near the required goal or optimum weight you want then slowly add more carbohydrates in the diet plan to slow down the further weight loss now.

2. Maintenance Phase (phase 4): Each as much carbs as much you can but

keep it in mind that the body shouldn't regain the weight. Excess of everything is bad.

A number of people skip the induction phase and intake lots of fruits and vegetables at the beginning that can be effective too. Other do prefer induction phase to activate ketosis process which is low-carb keto diet.

Foods for Atkins Diet:

People usually get confused what should be eating during the diet and what should not... an outlines of food is listed below:

Prohibited food:

Try to avoid the mentioned food items while you are on the Atkins diet plan:

Grains: Spelt, rye, Wheat, barley, rice.

Sugar: Fruit juices, cakes, Soft drinks, candy, ice cream, etc

Vegetable Oils: Soybean oil, cottonseed oil, corn oil, canola oil and many others.

Low-Fat Foods: foods those are rich in sugar content.

Trans Fats: The tin pack things with mentioning of hydrogenated ingredients on the list.

High-Carb Fruits: Apples, oranges, pears, bananas, grapes (while in induction phase).

Starches: Sweet potatoes, Potatoes (for induction phase only).

High-Carb Vegetables: Turnips, Carrots, etc (for induction only).

Legumes: Lentils, chickpeas, beans.

Beneficial Food items:

Healthy food items like the following should be in your menu for the Atkins diet Seafood and Fatty Fish: Trout, Salmon, sardines, etc.

Meats: Lamb, chicken, Beef, pork, bacon and others.

Eggs: Eggs are rich in Omega-3.

Healthy Fats: Coconut oil, avocado oil and extra virgin olive oil.

Full-Fat Dairy: Butter, full-fat yoghurt, cheese, cream.

Low-Carb Vegetables: Spinach, broccoli, Kale, asparagus and others alike.

Nuts and Seeds: Macadamia nuts, sunflower seeds, almonds, walnuts, etc.

Recipes

1. Blue Cheese and Bacon Soup

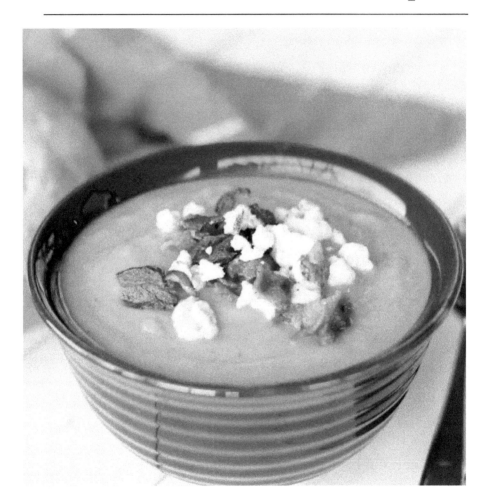

Ingredients:

- 6 strips of bacon
- 3 tbsp.butter

- 2 cups button, cremini, Portobello, or shitake mushrooms (sliced)
- 2 leeks (halved lengthwise then chopped)
- 1 ½ cups cauliflower florets
- 29 oz. chicken broth
- ½ cup of water
- 5 oz. blue cheese (crumbled)

Directions:

1. Heat a skillet over medium-high heat. Cook 3 strips of bacon until crispy on one side. Turn the bacon over and cook until crispy all over. Remove from pan and place on a plate with paper towels to remove any excess fat.

2. Do the same with the remaining bacon strips. Set aside and let it cool.

3. Meanwhile, put butter in a soup pot and let it melt over medium heat. Add the mushrooms, leek and cauliflower. Cover pot and let it cook for 5 minutes; stir vegetables occasionally.

4. Add chicken broth and water. Bring soup to a boil, leaving pot uncovered.

5. Lower heat and cover pot. Let soup simmer for 10 minutes or until vegetables turn very tender.

6. Puree the soup in batches using a food processor or a blender until smooth. On the last batch of soup, add blue cheese and puree.

7. Put the soup back in pot and heat if necessary.

8. Take cooked bacon and crumble. Serve the soup hot and sprinkle with crumbled bacon.

2. Spicy Tuna Steak Salad

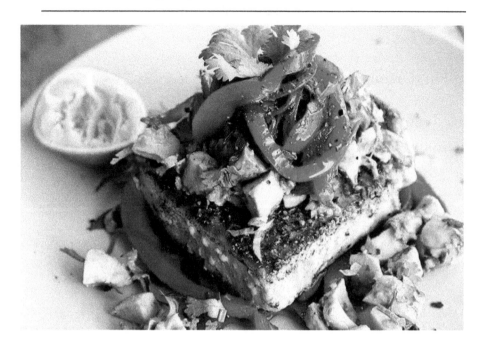

Ingredients:

- 2 tbsp. lemon zest
- 2 tsp. coriander (ground)
- 2 tsp. salt
- 1 ½ tsp. black pepper (freshly ground)
- 1 ½ tsp. ginger (ground)
- ½ tsp. cinnamon
- 1 ½ lbs. tuna (4 steaks)
- 4 tbsp. extra virgin olive oil
- 2 tps. balsamic vinegar
- 2 cups arugula

Directions:

1. In a small bowl, combine the lemon zest, coriander, salt, pepper, ginger and cinnamon. Add 2 tablespoons of the olive oil and stir thoroughly. Rub the mixture on the tuna steaks.

2. In a large skillet, heat 1 tbsp. of oil over high heat. Sauté the tuna steaks for 2-3 minutes, turn and cook for another 2-3 minutes until tuna is just cooked through.

3. Meanwhile, on a separate small bowl, place the balsamic vinegar and whisk in 1 tablespoon (or more, if desired) of olive oil. Add salt and pepper and continue to whisk mixture until a slightly thick dressing is made.

4. Toss arugula with the dressing until evenly coated.

5. Slice the tuna into ¼-inch pieces and serve over salad greens.

3. Athenian Salad

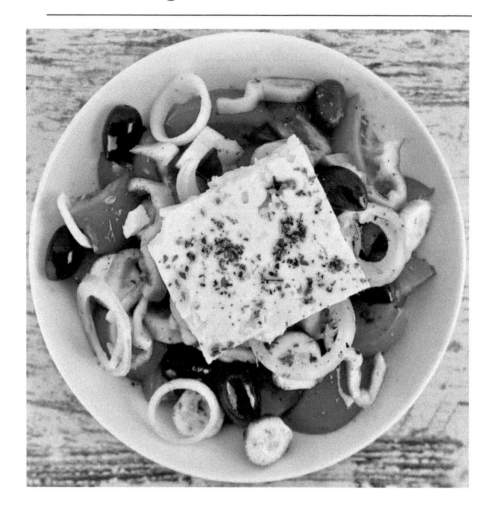

Ingredients:

- 6 Tbsp extra-virgin olive oil
- 1 clove garlic, finely minced
- 1½ tsp dried oregano, crumbled, or 1 Tbsp fresh oregano, chopped
- ½ tsp salt

- ¼ tsp freshly ground black pepper
- 2 Tbsp + 1 tsp freshly squeezed lemon juice
- ½ small red onion, thinly sliced
- 1½ medium cucumbers, peeled, halved lengthwise, seeded, and thinly sliced
- 1 medium green bell pepper, stemmed, ribs removed, and thinly sliced
- ½ cup pitted quartered kalamata or other black olives
- 12 cherry tomatoes, quartered
- ½ cup crumbled feta cheese

Instructions:

1.Whisk together oil, garlic, oregano, salt and pepper in a small bowl; whisk in lemon juice.

2.Put onion, cucumbers, bell pepper, and olives in a bowl and toss with the dressing. Arrange on a large platter or four individual plates, top with tomatoes and cheese, and serve.

4. Caprese Salad

Ingredients:

- 1 pound fresh mozzarella, cut into ¼-inch slices
- 4 medium tomatoes, cored and cut into ¼-inch slices
- ¼ cup extra-virgin olive oil
- 4 tsp red wine vinegar
- 1 tsp granular sugar substitute
- ½ tsp salt
- ¼ tsp freshly ground black pepper
- 6 basil leaves, cut into thin strips

Instructions:

1. Arrange mozzarella and tomatoes on a platter, alternating and overlapping the slices decoratively.
2. Whisk together oil, vinegar, sugar substitute, salt, and pepper in a small bowl.
3. Drizzle over cheese and tomatoes, and then scatter basil on top.

5. Old Bay Shrimp Salad

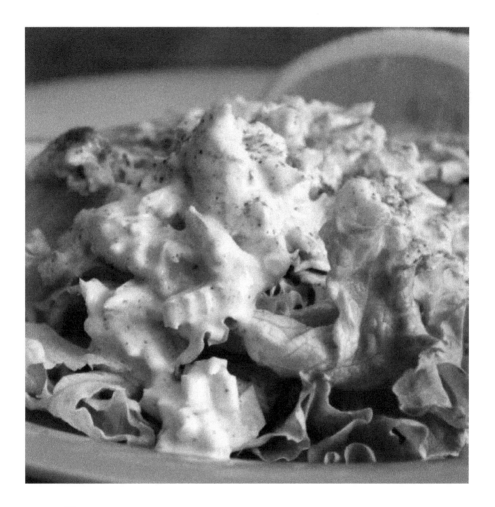

Ingredients:

- 1 pound frozen cooked small shrimp, defrosted
- 1 cup cauliflower florets, chopped
- 2 celery stalks, thinly sliced
- ¾ cup mayonnaise

- 2 scallions, thinly sliced
- 1 Tbsp Old Bay seasoning or seasoning salt
- 1 head Bibb lettuce, broken into 12 leaves

Instructions:

1. Drain the shrimp on paper towels or a kitchen towel to be sure they are dry.
2. Transfer to a bowl along with the cauliflower, celery, mayonnaise, scallions, and Old Bay.
3. Stir well.
4. Set the leaves out on salad plates and divide the salad among the 12 leaves and serve immediately

6. Watercress Bacon Salad with Ranch Dressing

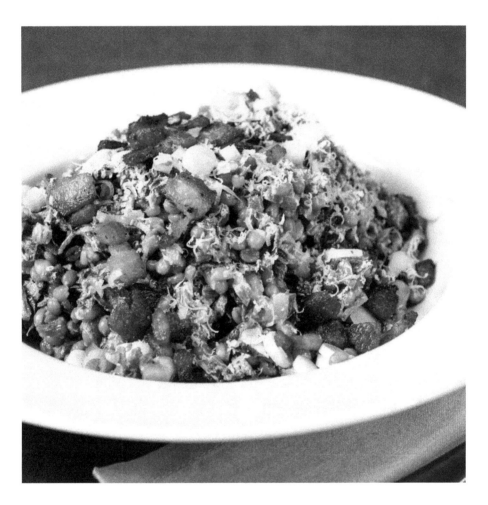

Ingredients:

- ½ pound watercress
- ½ pound baby spinach

- 2 tomatoes, chopped
- 1 ripe Hass avocado, diced
- 4 slices cooked bacon, crumbled

Ranch Dressing

- ½ cup mayonnaise
- 2 Tbsp canned coconut milk or heavy cream
- 1 tsp apple cider vinegar
- ½ tsp onion powder
- ½ tsp garlic salt
- 1 Tbsp chopped fresh dill or flat-leaf parsley
- ¼ tsp freshly ground black pepper

Instructions:

1.Combine the watercress and spinach, tossing well. Put equally on four plates and top with the tomatoes, avocado, and bacon.

2.Place the mayonnaise, coconut milk or heavy cream, vinegar, onion powder, garlic salt, dill or parsley, and black pepper in a large bowl.

3.Whisk well to combine. Serve over the salad.

7. Chicken, Mushrooom And Bok Choy Soup

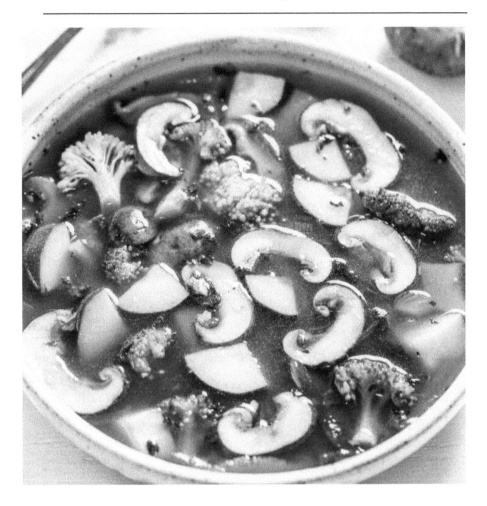

Ingredients:

- 43.5 oz chicken broth
- 3 tbsp. ginger root, shopped finely
- 12 oz. shiitake mushrooms

- 4 tbsp. Nam Pla fish sauce
- 2 tbsp. tamari
- 1 tbsp. sesame oil
- 1/8 tsp. red pepper flakes (crushed)
- 10 oz. chicken (breast part, shredded)
- ¾ lbs. bok choy (sliced)
- 4 tsp. rice vinegar (unsweetened)
- 2 medium-sized green onions (sliced thinly)

Directions:

1. In a large pot, pour in chicken broth and add ginger and mushrooms. Bring to a boil. Lower the heat and let it simmer for 3 minutes.

2. Add the Nam Pla fish sauce, tamari, sesame oil and pepper flakes. Let it simmer for 2 more minutes.

3. Add the shredded chicken and bok choy, then let it simmer for another 2 minutes.

4. Stir in the rice vinegar and add salt and pepper to taste.

5. Remove from heat and serve garnished with green onion slices.

8. Chicken Bacon Club Salad

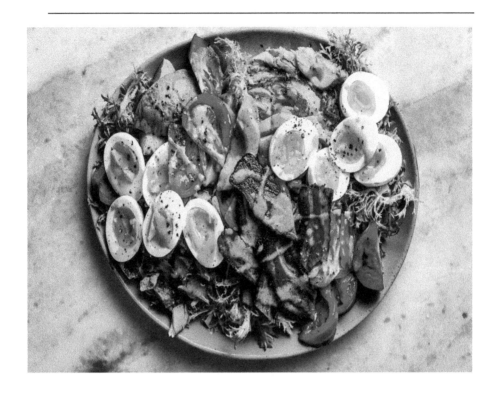

Ingredients:

- 4 boneless skinless chicken breasts
- 1 Cup Mayo
- 6 slices bacon
- 2 Cups shredded cheddar cheese

Directions:

1. Cook bacon until crisp, then crumble.
2. Cube chicken breast and cook thoroughly.
3. Mix all ingredients together.

4. Spared into a 8" cake pan.

5. Bake for about 15 minutes.

6. Serve on top of a bed of lettuce. Top with black olives if you like.

9. Chicken Taco Salad

Ingredients:

- 4 chicken breast – boil, then shred with fork
- Olive Oil Cumin
- Chili Powder 1 Can Rotel tomatoes with green chilis
- 1 Large yellow onion – diced 1 Head Iceberg lettuce
- 1 Can black olives Shredded cheddar cheese
- Sour Cream Guacamole (optional)Homemade Salsa:
- 1 large can peeled tomatoes 1 small bunch cilantro
- 1 medium/large onion garlic salt

Directions:

1. In a large skillet, pour about 2 Tblsp olive oil and turn up to med/high heat. Sautee about ¼ of the onions.
2. Add the shredded chicken, cumin and chili powder and Rotel.
3. Simmer for approximately 20 minutes, stirring occasionally. Meanwhile, shred lettuce and place in bowls.
4. When Chicken mixture is done, place a heaping on top of the lettuce and cover with cheese, olives, sour cream, the remaining onions.
5. Combine salsa ingredients in blender.
6. Add to salad this will be used as your dressing.

10.   Easy Egg Plant Salad

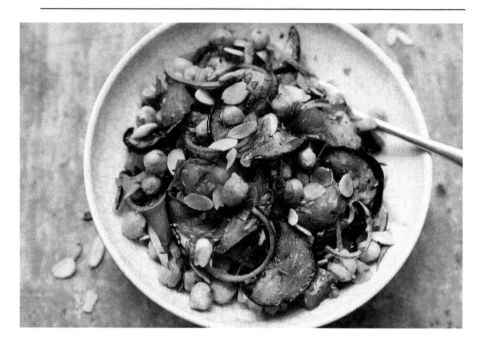

Ingredients:

- 1 large eggplant – cut
- ½" pieces 1 large onion – cut
- ½" pieces, (red, white, yellow, spanish)
- 1 can pitted black olives – diced small
- 1 small jar spanish olives diced into small pieces
- ¼ cup cider vinegar – more to taste
- 1 quart tomato sauce – whatever low carb brand you use

Directions:

1. Mix all chopped ingredients and add the vinegar. Toss well to mix the vinegar with the mixed veggies. Let set a few minutes and toss again. Add the tomato sauce and mix again.

2. Add red pepper and black to taste (1/2 tsp red is hot). Mix one more time before placing in a 4 qt.

3. Corning ware pot. Bake in the oven at 325`F for about 1 hour (1 ½ hours is mushy)

4. Let cool to room temperature, toss and refigerate before serving (sandwich spread, appetizer, main course with chicken,pork or beef).

5. recipe is about 15 minutes, has a very unique taste that satisfies the appetite.

11.   Chilled Seafood Bisque

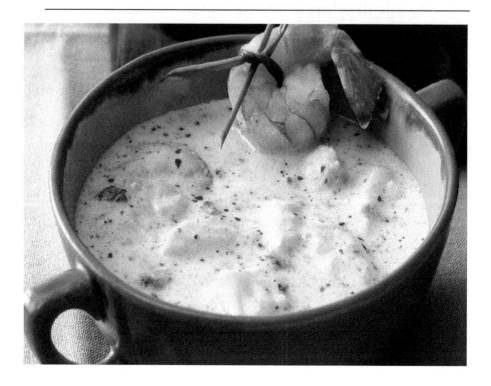

Ingredients:

- 1 tbsp. butter (unsalted)
- 1/3 cup medium-sized white onion (chopped)
- 27 oz. clam juice
- ¾ cup heavy cream
- 1/8 tbsp. thyme
- 6 pcs. Large shrimps (cooked and diced)

Directions:

1. Place a saucepan over medium-low heat and melt butter. Cook onions for 3 to 4 minutes, or until they turn translucent.

2. Pour in the clam juice and bring to a boil. Reduce heat slightly, cook for 5 minutes and let it cool.

3. Meanwhile, in a separate small saucepan, mix in cream and thyme and bring to a boil. Reduce heat slightly and cook for 5 to 7 minutes, or until mixture is reduced to just about half a cup. Discard thyme and let it cool.

4. Stir in reduced cream to the clam juice and puree mixture in batches using a food processor or blender until smooth.

5. Place in an airtight container and chill in the fridge until just cool or cold, depending on your preference.

6. Serve in four bowls then top with diced shrimps. Garnish with a small sprig of thyme if desired.

12.   Creamy Spinach Soup

Ingredients:

- 2 tbsp. butter (unsalted)
- 1 pc. of small onion (chopped finely)
- 1 tsp. garlic (chopped)
- 43 ½ oz. chicken broth
- 20 oz. frozen chopped spinach (thawed)
- 2 cups heavy cream
- 1/2tsp. ground nutmeg

Directions:

1. Place a large stockpot over medium heat and melt butter. Sauté onions for about 4 minutes or until they turn soft. Add in the garlic and sauté for about 30 seconds until aroma is released.

2. Add the broth and spinach then let it simmer for around 5 minutes. Remove from heat.

3. Puree the soup in batches using a food processor or a blender until smooth. Put soup back in the pot and add the cream. Cook over low heat until soup is warm.

4. Stir in nutmeg and remove from heat. Season with salt and pepper to taste and serve.

13. Tarragon Shrimp Salad

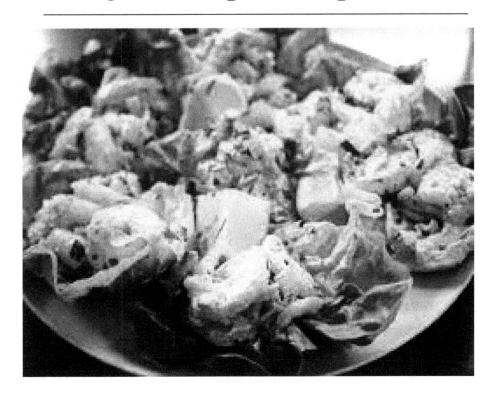

Ingredients:

- ¼ cup mayonnaise
- 2 tbsp. Dijon mustard
- 2 tbsp. dried capers
- 1 tbsp. fresh parsley (chopped)
- 1 tsp. fresh tarragon (chopped)
- 2 anchovy fillets (oil-packed, mashed)
- 1 ½ lbs. medium-sized shrimps (deveined, cooked and shelled)

Directions:

1. Whisk together all ingredients except for the shrimp in a large serving bowl. Mix well until evenly combined. Add salt and pepper to taste.

2. Add the shrimp and toss well so that shrimp is evenly coated. Serve immediately

14.   Turkey Cobb Salad with Italian Dressing

Ingredients:

For Salad:

- 6 bacon strips
- 6 cups Romaine lettuce (shredded)
- 2 large eggs (hard-boiled, peeled, diced)
- 2 cups turkey (cooked, chopped)
- 1 hass avocado (cubed)
- 2 small tomatoes (cored, chopped)
- ¾ cup blue cheese (crumbled)

For Italian Dressing:

- ½ cup extra virgin olive oil
- 1 medium clove of garlic (pressed or finely minced)
- 2 tbsp. red wine vinegar
- 1 ½ tbsp. fresh parsley (minced)
- 1 tbsp. lemon juice (freshly squeezed)
- ½ tbsp. fresh basil (minced)
- 1 tsp. dried oregano
- ¼ tsp. red pepper flakes

- ½ tsp. granular sugar substitute (sucralose)
- 1/8 tsp. salt
- 1/8 tsp. freshly ground pepper.

Directions:

1. First prepare the dressing by combining all ingredients with a blender. Set aside or refrigerate if desired.

2. On a skillet, cook bacon over medium-high heat until crispy. Drain off excess fat with a paper towel and chop coarsely or crumble with hands when cool enough. Set aside.

3. In a large bowl, toss the Romaine lettuce with around 3 tablespoons of the Italian dressing. Place lettuce on a large serving platter.

4. Place the remaining salad ingredients over the lettuce, arranging them in vertical stripes if you wish.

5. Drizzle with remaining Italian dressing and serve immediately.

15.   Guacamole Soup

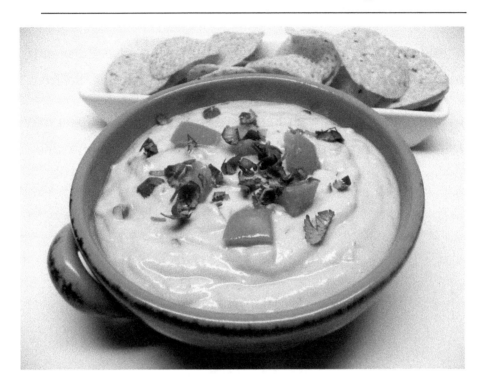

Ingredients:

- 2 medium-sized green onions (cut into 1-in pcs)
- ½ cup fresh cilantro leaves
- 1 pc. fresh jalapeno (seeded, chopped coarsely)
- 2 hass avocado (peeled, pitted, chopped coarsely)
- 14 ½ oz. chicken broth
- ½ cup tomato juice
- ¼ cup lemon juice

Directions:

1. Using a food processor, pulse onions, cilantro leaves and jalapeno until mixture is finely chopped.

2. Add avocado, broth, tomato juice and lemon juice. Pulse until mixture is smooth. Season with salt, and add Tabasco if desired.

3. Refrigerate for an hour and serve chilled. If desired, you may prepare the soup 8 hours ahead and let it chill overnight to allow flavors to blend well.

16.   Quick Bouillabaisse

Ingredients:

- ¼ cup extra virgin olive oil
- 2 stalks of celery (chopped)
- ½ small fennel bulb (chopped)
- ½ small onion (chopped)
- 1 garlic clove (sliced thinly)
- 29 oz. chicken broth
- 14 ½ oz. water
- 3 tbsp. orange zest (or 3 strips of 2 x ½ in orange peel)
- 2 tbsp. tomato paste
- ½ tsp. fennel seeds
- ½ tsp. dried tarragon
- 20 mussels (washed and beards pulled off)
- 1 ½ lbs. fish fillets (white fish like snapper, cod, or monk fish; cut into 2 pieces)
- 1 lb. medium-sized shrimps (shelled)
- ¼ cup fresh parsley (chopped)

Directions:

1.In a large saucepot, heat the olive oil over medium heat. Add the celery, fennel and onion then cook for around 5 minutes, until they soften. Add the garlic and cook for another minute.

2.Pour in the chicken broth and water. Add the orange zest (or peel), tomato paste, fennel seeds and tarragon. Bring to a boil.

3.Reduce the heat and add the mussels. Cover pot and cook for 10 minutes.

4.Add the fish fillet. Wait for 5 minutes then add the shrimp. Cook for 35 more minutes. Season with salt and freshly ground pepper to taste. 5.Divide in serving bowls. Make sure that you discard any unopened mussels, if any. Garnish with parsley and serve hot.

17.   Broccoli, Olives, & Egg Salad

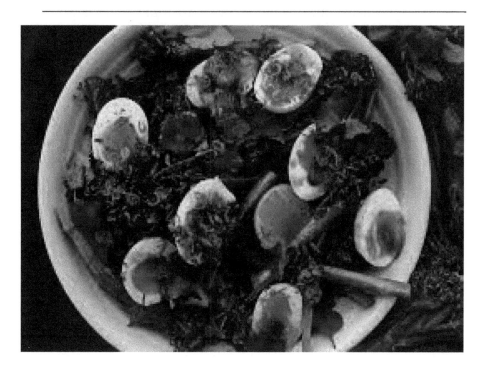

Ingredients:

- Fresh broccoli florets Boiled eggs
- Green olives Red Onion
- Mayonnaise Black Pepper
- Paprika Salt

Directions:

1. Quantities of everything according to taste.
2. I would use I bunch broccoli, 3 eggs chopped in large pieces, ½ cup olives, ½ large red onion chopped.

3. The rest of the ingredients really depend on your preferences, but black pepper really makes this salad.
4. Mix everything together and coat well with mayo.
5. Chill and serve.

18.　Bruschetta Style Tomato Turkey Salad

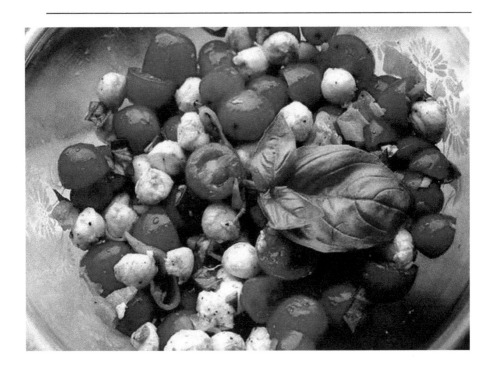

Ingredients:

- 1 cup ground turkey 1 cup mixed lettuce
- 1 tomato
- 4 or 5 kalamata olives
- salt pepper
- 1 or 2 T olive oil
- 1 tsp crushed garlic 1 tsp basil paste (or a few leaves of finely chopped fresh basil)

Directions:

1. Dice the tomato and place in a small bowl.
2. Add chopped olives, olive oil, garlic, basil, and salt and pepper to taste.
3. Brown the turkey mince in a saucepan.
4. Add the tomato mix to the turkey and mix together.
5. Serve over a bed of mixed lettuce.

19.   Caulif-broccoli salad

Ingredients:

- 1 lg head cauliflower
- 1 lg bunch broccoli
- 1 sm onion (or 4 green ones)
- 1 pkg froz peas (or pea pods)
- 2 cups mayo
- 1 cup sour cream 1 tsp garlic powder

Directions:

1. Mix mayo, sour cream and garlic powder in a small bowl.
2. Break caulif and broccoli into bite sized florets.
3. Add onion.
4. Toss sauce with broccoli, cauliflower and onion.
5. Add peas last (if using pods, cut into ¼ inch pieces). Refrigerate at least 4 hours or overnight.

20.   Jalapeño Cheddar Broccoli Soup

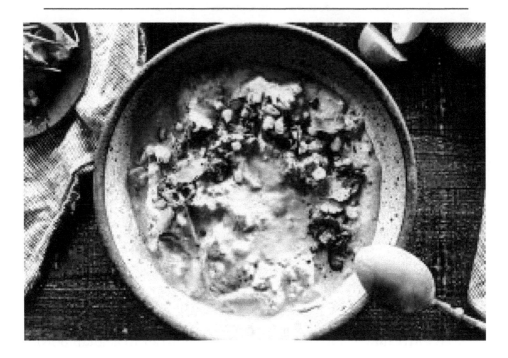

Ingredients:

- 3 Tbsp olive oil
- 1 head broccoli, cut into florets
- 6 jalapeños, seeded and diced
- ½ onion, chopped
- 1 tsp salt
- ½ tsp curry powder or ground turmeric
- ½ tsp freshly ground black pepper
- 2 Tbsp flour
- 1 quart bone broth, or unsalted chicken or beef broth

- ¼ cup heavy cream
- 1 Tbsp hot sauce
- 4 slices (4 ounces) cheddar cheese

Instructions:

1. Warm the olive oil in a stockpot.
2. Add the broccoli, jalapeños, onion, salt, curry powder or turmeric, and pepper; cook 5 to 6 minutes, stirring often, until the onion begins to brown.
3. Sprinkle with the flour and cook 1 minute more, stirring often, until the flour coats the vegetables. Add the broth and cover.
4. Cook for 15 minutes.
5. Using an immersion blender, blend until smooth. Stir in the heavy cream and hot sauce.
6. Set the oven to broil. Transfer the soup to four oven-safe bowls and top each with one a slice of cheese.
7. Place under the broiler for 3 minutes, until the cheese is melted and bubbly. Serve immediately.

21.   Cauliflower Bisque

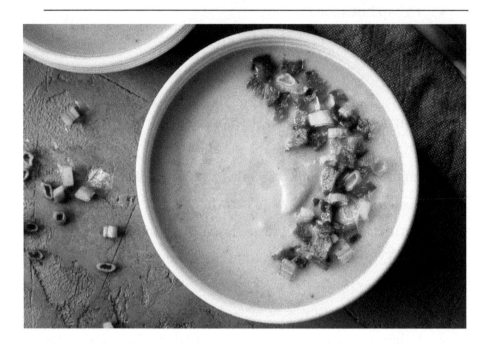

Ingredients:

- 3 tablespoons unsalted butter
- 1 head cauliflower, cut into florets
- 4 garlic cloves, chopped
- ½ teaspoon salt
- ½ teaspoon freshly grated nutmeg
- ¼ teaspoon freshly ground black pepper
- 1 quart basic bone broth or unsalted chicken or vegetable broth
- 1 tablespoon lemon juice
- ½ cup heavy cream or canned coconut milk

- 4 teaspoons olive oil
- ½ red bell pepper, minced

Instructions:

1. Put the butter in a large stockpot, and warm over medium heat, about 1 minute, until the butter foams.
2. Add the cauliflower, garlic, salt, nutmeg, and pepper; cook 5 to 6 minutes, stirring often, until the garlic begins to brown.
3. Add the broth and lemon juice and cover.
4. Cook 15 to 20 minutes, until the cauliflower is fork tender.
5. Using an immersion blender, blend until smooth.
6. Stir in the heavy cream or coconut milk.
7. Spoon into 4 bowls, garnish each serving with the olive oil and bell pepper, and serve immediately.

22.   Spicy Korean Soup with Scallions

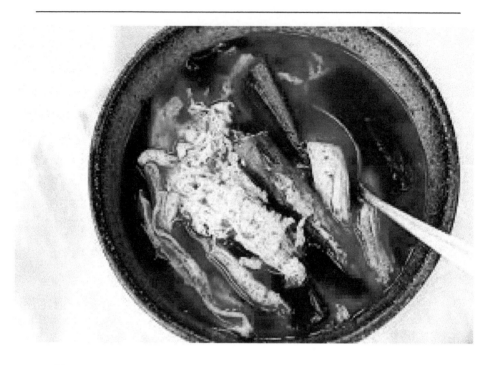

Ingredients:

- 1 pound flank steak
- ½ tsp freshly ground black pepper
- 3 Tbsp sesame oil
- 10 ounces mushrooms, such as button, shiitake, or cremini
- 8 scallions, thinly sliced
- 4 garlic cloves, minced
- 2 tsp crushed red pepper flakes
- ¼ tsp salt

- 2 Tbsp soy sauce or tamari
- 2 Tbsp apple cider vinegar
- 1 quart beef broth

Instructions:

1. Place the flank steak in a large stockpot, and cover with water.
2. Add the black pepper and bring to a boil over high heat. Reduce the heat to low and simmer, covered, for 2 hours, until the meat is very tender.
3. Drain, discarding the liquid, and let the beef cool. Use a fork to shred the meat.
4. Wash and dry the stockpot. Warm the oil in the stockpot over medium-low heat.
5. Add the mushrooms, scallions, garlic, red pepper flakes, and salt, and cook for about 3 minutes, stirring often, until fragrant.
6. Add the shredded beef, soy sauce or tamari, vinegar, and broth.
7. Bring to a simmer and cook for 5 minutes, until the mushrooms are tender.
8. Serve immediately.

23.   Caesar Salad

Ingredients:

- 1 head Romaine lettuce (torn into bite-size pcs.)
- 7 tbsp. parmesan cheese (grated)
- ¼ cup mayonnaise
- 1 tbsp. fresh lemon juice
- 1 tbsp. extra virgin olive oil
- 1 tbsp. anchovy paste
- 1 ½ tsp. Worcestershire sauce
- 1 tsp. Dijon mustard
- 1 tsp. garlic (minced finely)
- ¼ tsp. salt
- ¼ tsp. freshly ground black pepper
- 1/8 tbsp. Tabasco (optional)
- 8 canned anchovies (drained, optional)

Directions:

1.Place lettuce and 4 tablespoons of the cheese in a large bowl and toss.

2.To make dressing, combine all remaining ingredients, except for anchovies, in a small bowl.

3.Toss in mixture with the lettuce until the dressing is evenly distributed.

4.Serve in four separate plates and top with 2 anchovies each, if desired.

24. Canned Tuna And Artichoke Salad

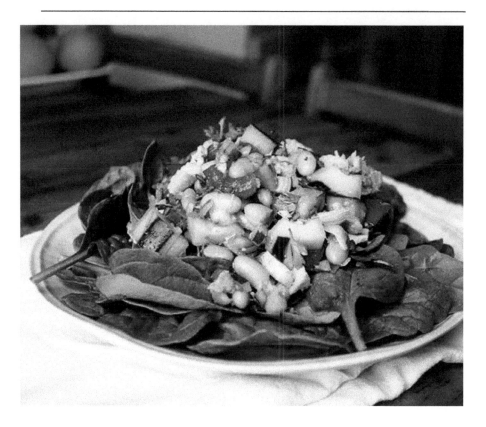

Ingredients:

- 4 oz. canned tuna
- 3 pcs. Marinated artichoke hearts (chopped)
- 2 tbsp. mayonnaise
- 2 cups Romaine lettuce (shredded)

Directions:

1.Drain canned tuna. Place tuna in a mixing bowl and combine with artichoke and mayonnaise. Season with salt and ground pepper.

2.Assemble lettuce on a plate. Top with tuna mixture and serve.

25.   Chef Salad With Blue Cheese Dressing

Ingredients:

For Salad

- 1 strip of bacon
- 6 oz. chicken breast
- 1 cup mixed greens
- ½ hass avocado (sliced)
- ½ medium-sized tomato (chopped)
- ¼ cup Monterey Jack cheese (diced)

For Blue Cheese Dressing:

- 4 oz. blue cheese (crumbled)
- ½ cup sour cream
- ½ cup mayonnaise
- 1/3 cup heavy cream
- 1 tbsp. fresh lemon juice
- ½ tsp. Dijon mustard
- ½ tsp. freshly ground pepper

Directions:

1.Cook bacon until crispy on a skillet over medium-high heat. Drain off excess fat on a paper towel and let it stand for a while until cool enough to crumble. Set aside.

2.Poach the chicken in water set over medium heat. Cook for around 8 minutes, until meat turns white. Remove chicken from water and chop into bitesized pieces. Sprinkle with salt and pepper to taste.

3.Prepare Blue Cheese Dressing by combining the ingredients in a medium bowl. Use a fork to break up the cheese and mash the mixture until combined well.

4.Place salad greens, avocado, tomato and Monterey Jack cheese in the same bowl and toss well until evenly coated with dressing. Sprinkle with crumbled bacon and serve.

26.   Salsa Verde Chicken Soup

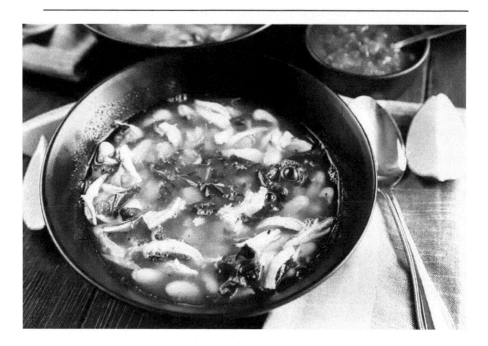

Ingredients:

- 4 chicken breasts, on the bone, skin intact (about 1½ pounds)
- ½ tsp salt
- ½ tsp mild chili powder
- ¼ tsp freshly ground black pepper
- 2 Tbsp olive oil
- ½ red or white onion, minced
- 2 cups cauliflower florets
- 2 cups fresh cilantro leaves and stems, chopped and divided

- 4 garlic cloves
- 1 quart unsalted chicken broth
- ½ cup commercial salsa verde
- ¼ cup sour cream

Instructions:

1. Sprinkle the chicken with the salt, chili powder, and pepper. Warm the oil in a stockpot over medium heat.
2. Add the chicken and cook for 8 minutes, turning a few times, until the chicken is well browned. Transfer the chicken to a plate.
3. Add the onion, cauliflower, half the cilantro, and the garlic, cooking 5 to 6 minutes more, until the vegetables soften.
4. Return the chicken to the stockpot, and cover with the broth.
5. Bring to a simmer and cook 20 to 25 minutes, until the chicken is cooked through.
6. Remove the skin and bones.
7. Shred the chicken.
8. Return it to the soup, and top with the salsa verde and the remaining cilantro.
9. Serve with the sour cream.

27.   Chicken Vegetable Soup

Ingredients:

- 1 pound skinless chicken breasts
- ½ cup chopped carrots
- ¼ cup chopped celery
- ¼ cup chopped onion
- Salt and pepper

Instructions:

1. Cook chicken breasts in a pot with 2½ cups of water over medium heat for 20 minutes.

2. Remove the chicken from the broth and cut into strips.

3. Put the chicken strips back into the pot with the broth.

4. Season with salt and pepper.

5. Add the rest of the ingredients.

6. Cook for about 1 hour more or until vegetables are done.

28.   Thai Coconut-Shrimp Soup

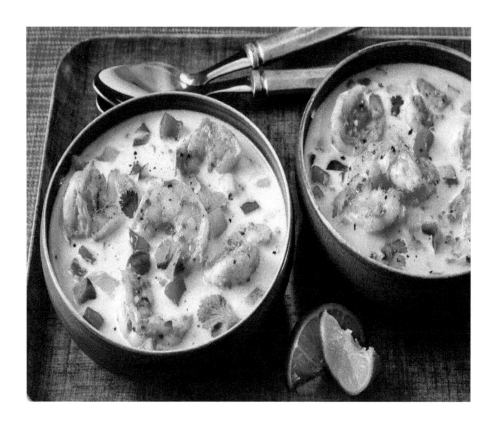

Ingredients:

- 3 cups chicken broth
- 1 (13½-ounce) can unsweetened coconut milk
- 1 (1-inch) piece fresh ginger, peeled, cut into ⅛-inch slices
- 2 Tbsp fish sauce (nam pla or nuoc nam)
- 1 jalapeño, finely chopped
- 1 Tbsp freshly grated lime zest

- 1 tsp granular sugar substitute
- 1 pound medium shrimp, peeled and deveined
- 4 ounces button mushrooms, cut into ¼-inch slices (optional)
- 2 scallions, thinly sliced
- ¼ cup chopped fresh cilantro
- 1 Tbsp fresh lime juice

Instructions:

1. Combine first seven ingredients in a soup pot over medium-low heat. Bring to a low boil and simmer for 10 minutes.

2. Add shrimp and mushrooms, if using; simmer until shrimp are cooked through, 3 to 5 minutes.

3.Remove and discard ginger.

4.Stir in the remaining 3 ingredients and serve.

29. Chinese Hot-and-Sour Soup

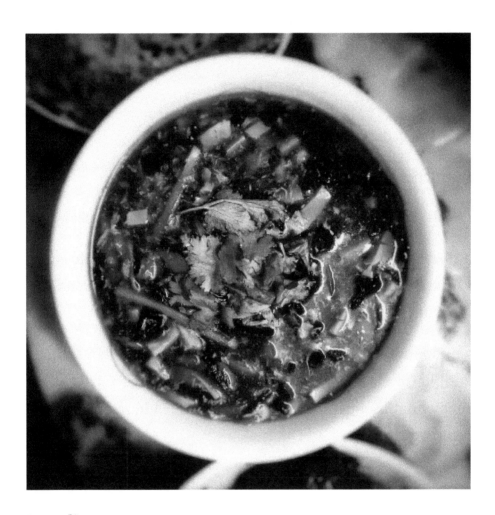

Ingredients:

- ⅓ cup unseasoned, unsweetened rice vinegar
- 1 Tbsp Dixie Carb Counters Thick-It-Up low-carb thickener
- 1 tsp canola oil

- 1 clove garlic, finely chopped
- ½ cup button mushrooms, thinly sliced
- 4 cups chicken broth
- 1 (10½-ounce) package firm tofu, cut into ¼-inch dice
- 2 Tbsp tamari
- ½ tsp red pepper flakes
- 1 tsp dark (toasted) sesame oil

Instructions:

1.Whisk together vinegar and thickener in a small bowl; set aside.

2.Heat canola oil in a soup pot over medium-high heat. Add garlic and sauté until fragrant, about 30 seconds. Add mushrooms and sauté until slightly soft, about 3 minutes.

3.Add broth, tofu, tamari, and pepper flakes; cover and simmer until flavors blend, 5 to 7 minutes. Stir in vinegar mixture and simmer until soup thickens, about 1 minute. Add sesame oil just before serving.

30. Creamy Cheddar Cheese Soup

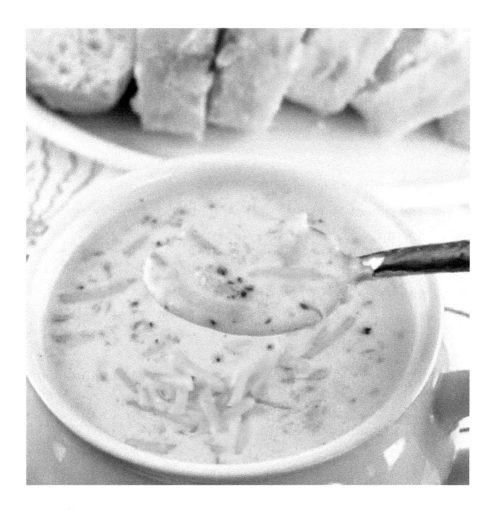

Ingredients:

- 1 Tbsp butter
- 1 shallot, minced
- 2½ cups vegetable broth

- 1 Tbsp Dixie Carb Counters Thick-It-Up low-carb thickener
- 1½ cups half-and-half
- 8 ounces Cheddar cheese, shredded (2 cups)
- 2 tsp hot paprika
- ½ tsp salt

Instructions:

1. Melt butter in a saucepan.
2. Add shallot and sauté until soft, about 3 minutes.
3. Add broth and bring to a simmer.
4. Whisk in thickener; cook until mixture thickens, about 2 minutes.
5. Add half-and-half and simmer, stirring occasionally, until hot.
6. Slowly whisk in cheese until melted and thoroughly combined.
7. Stir in paprika and salt and serve.

31. Cream of Broccoli Soup

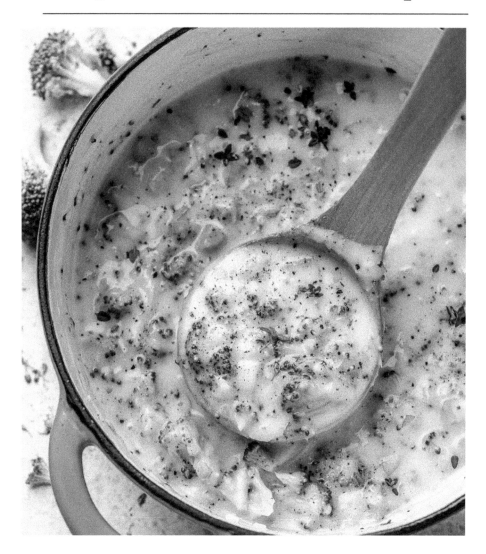

Ingredients:

- 4 cups vegetable or chicken broth
- 1 tsp salt
- ¼ tsp freshly ground black pepper

- 1 pound broccoli, cut into florets; stems peeled and cut into 1-inch pieces
- 1 Tbsp Dixie Carb Counters Thick-It-Up low-carb thickener
- 1 cup heavy cream

Instructions:

1. Combine broth, salt, and pepper in a soup pot over medium-high heat; bring to a boil.
2. Add broccoli, reduce the heat to medium-low, and simmer until tender, about 15 minutes.
3. Transfer soup to a blender.
4. Blend at low speed to purée. Return soup to the pot; bring back to a simmer over medium-high heat.
5. Whisk in thickener and cream; simmer, whisking occasionally, until thick and hot, about 5 minutes.
6. Serve hot or refrigerate in an airtight container for up to 3 days.
7. Reheat before serving.

32.   Cold Roasted Tomato Soup

Ingredients:

- 3 pounds fresh plum tomatoes, halved lengthwise
- 1 small yellow onion, peeled and quartered
- 3 Tbsp extra-virgin olive oil
- 3 cloves garlic, peeled
- 1½ tsp salt
- ½ tsp freshly ground black pepper
- 4 cups chicken broth
- 6 Tbsp thinly sliced fresh basil

Instructions:

1. Heat oven to 450°F. Line a jelly-roll pan with parchment paper or foil.

2. Combine tomatoes, onion, oil, garlic, salt, and pepper in a mixing bowl; toss to coat. Transfer ingredients to the pan, making sure to include all of the liquid and arranging tomatoes cut side down in a single layer.

3. Roast until tomato skins are puckered and browned, about 20 minutes, rotating pan once halfway through. Let cool.

4. Add garlic and roasted vegetables and any juices to a blender.

5. Holding down blender lid firmly with a folded kitchen towel, blend at low speed until slightly chunky (you may have to work in batches).

6. Add broth and pulse once to combine.

5. Refrigerate until ready to serve or at least 1 hour. Serve, topped with basil.

33. Shaved Fennel Salad with Lemon Dressing

Ingredients:

- ¼ pound green beans, cut into 1½-inch pieces
- ¼ cup extra-virgin olive oil
- 3 Tbsp freshly squeezed lemon juice
- 1 tsp freshly grated lemon zest
- 1 tsp red wine vinegar
- ½ tsp salt
- ½ tsp freshly ground black pepper
- ¼ tsp granular sugar substitute
- 2 medium fennel bulbs, cored, quartered lengthwise, and thinly sliced crosswise
- 2 Tbsp chopped fresh basil

Instructions:

1. In a pot, bBring well-salted water to a boil over high heat. Add green beans and cook for about 4 minutes. Drain; set aside.

2. Combine oil, lemon juice, lemon zest, vinegar, salt, pepper, and sugar substitute in a salad bowl.

3. Add green beans, fennel, and basil and combine; cover and refrigerate at least 30 minutes but no more than 3 hours to let flavors blend.

4. Stir gently before serving.

34. Cucumber-Dill Salad

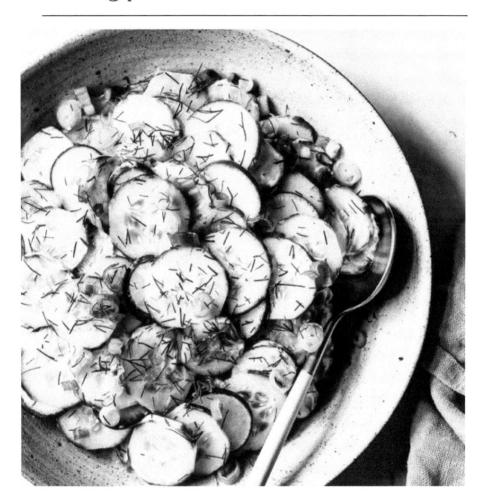

Ingredients:

- ½ cup white wine vinegar
- ¼ cup chopped fresh dill
- 2 tsp granular sugar substitute
- 1 tsp salt
- 4 medium cucumbers, thinly sliced

Instructions:

1. Combine vinegar, dill, sugar substitute, and salt in a medium bowl.

2. Add cucumbers and toss gently to coat.

3. Refrigerate 30 minutes to let flavors blend.

4. Drain excess liquid before serving.

35. Slaw with Vinegar Dressing

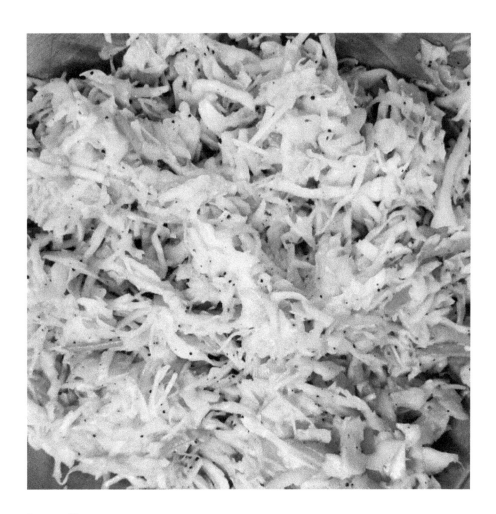

Ingredients:

- ⅓ cup white or red wine vinegar
- 1 Tbsp Dijon mustard
- 1 clove garlic, minced
- ⅓ cup extra-virgin olive oil

- ¼ cup chopped fresh parsley
- 4 small scallions, thinly sliced
- ½ tsp salt
- ½ tsp freshly ground black pepper
- ½ large head red or green cabbage, or a combination, shredded (8 cups)

Instructions:

1. Combine vinegar, mustard, and garlic in a salad bowl.

2. Add oil, whisking until dressing thickens.

3. Stir in parsley, scallions, salt, and pepper.

4. Add cabbage; toss to coat. Refrigerate for about 30 minutes before serving.

36. Wedge Salad with Gorgonzola Dressing

Ingredients:

- 4 romaine lettuce hearts
- 4 slices cooked bacon, crumbled
- 1 cup cherry or grape tomatoes, halved
- 2 cup beets, roasted or blanched, chilled, diced or cut into wedges
- 1 cup sliced radishes (or cucumber)

Gorgonzola Dressing

- ½ cup full-fat Greek yogurt
- ½ cup mayonnaise
- ¼ cup Gorgonzola, cut into small pieces
- 2 Tbsp lemon juice
- 1 tsp onion powder
- ½ tsp garlic salt
- ¼ tsp freshly ground black pepper
- ¼ tsp sweet paprika

Instructions:

To make the dressing, place the yogurt, mayonnaise, Gorgonzola, lemon juice, onion powder, garlic salt, pepper, and paprika in a medium bowl along with 2 tablespoons warm water and whisk well.

1. Refrigerate until ready to serve.
2. Fill two large bowls with lukewarm water.
3. Add the romaine hearts and soak 3 to 4 minutes while you prepare the dressing.
4. Drain the romaine, wrap in papertowels, and chill in the fridge for at least 1 hour to crisp it up.
5. Cut the romaine hearts in half and place two halves on each plate.
6. Drizzle with the dressing and sprinkle with pepper.
7. Top with the bacon, tomatoes, beets, radishes.
8. Serve with the remaining dressing.

37.   Tomato and Red Onion Salad

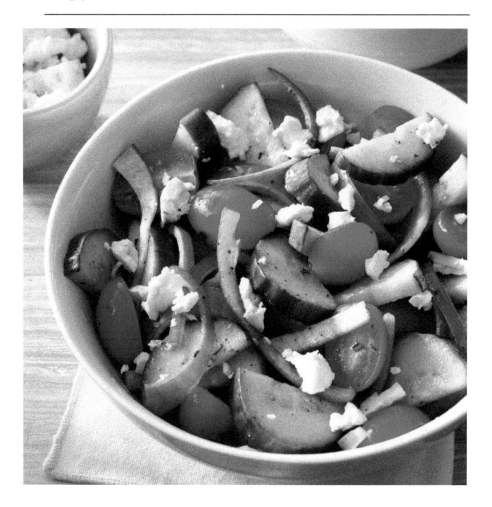

Ingredients:

- 3 Tbsp red wine vinegar
- 2 tsp Dijon mustard
- ¾ tsp salt
- ½ tsp freshly ground black pepper
- 5 Tbsp extra-virgin olive oil

- 3 large tomatoes, cut into 1-inch pieces
- ½ small red onion, thinly sliced
- ½ seedless cucumber, cut into ⅓-inch dice
- ¼ cup chopped fresh basil or dill
- 2 Tbsp capers, rinsed and drained

Instructions:

1.Combine first four ingredients in a salad bowl. Add oil, whisking until dressing thickens.

2.Add tomatoes, cucumbers, onion, basil, and capers; toss gently and serve right away.

38. Cream of Mushroom Soup

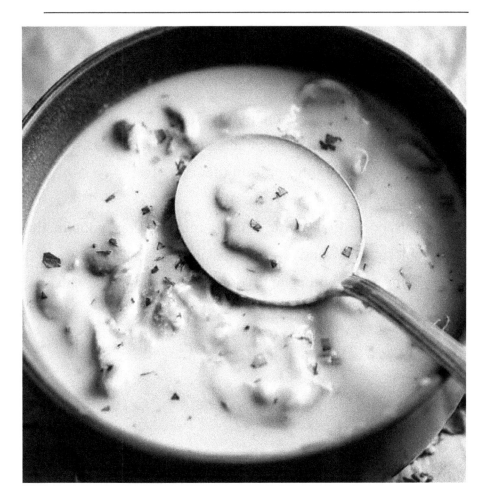

Ingredients:

- 8 ounces mushroom -- white button, finely chopped
- 1/4 cup chopped onion -- finely chopped
- 2 stalks celery -- finely chopped4 tablespoons butter
- 2 cups heavy cream
- 2 cans chicken stock

- 2 tablespoons flour
- 1 teaspoon salt
- 1/2 teaspoon pepper -- to taste

Directions:

1. In a large saucepan, melt butter over medium heat.
2. Add finely diced veggies and saute, stirring occasionally, for about 5 minutes or until they wilt.
3. Add in the flour and stir well.
4. Let cook, stirring, for about 1 minute, then pour in the chicken stock and cream, whisking constantly.
5. Bring to a simmer and cook about 5 minutes, whisking occasionally.

39.　Easy Chicken Noodle Soup

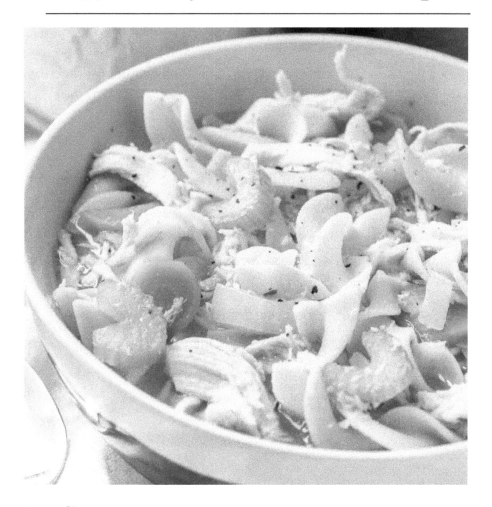

Ingredients:

- 2 tablespoons butter
- 1/4 onion
- 2 stalks celery
- 5 baby carrots
- 14 1/2 ounces chicken broth -- 1 can

- 10 ounces canned chicken -- 1 can
- Salt and Pepper to taste
- 1 teaspoon Wylers Shaker Instant Bouilion
- Chicken Garlic and Herb flavor or 1 chicken bouillon cube
- 1/2 package shiratake noodles

Directions:

1. Chop onion,celery and carrots. Brown them in the butter for a few min.
2. Add the broth, chicken, noodles and seasoning.
3. Bring to boil and then turn down and simmer for a few min.
4. I can get 4 or 5 good size servings.
5. You can add green bean, zucchini as well.

40.   Ground Beef Soup

Ingredients:

- 1 pound ground beef
- 1 cup diced onion
- 1 diced green bell pepper
- 8 cups beef stock
- 2 cups diced carrots -- i used 1 cup
- 1 cup diced celery
- 2 cups chopped tomatoes
- 1/4 cup minced fresh parsley1 package broccoli, frozen -- cut into
- florets
- or 1 head cut into floretswith stalks
- peeled and diced
- 1 teaspoon dried oregano
- 1 teaspoon dried thyme
- freshly ground black pepper to taste

Directions:

1. In large non-stick skillet, sauté; ground beef over medium heat.

2. Add onions, garlic and bell pepper and continue sautéing until meat is tender and vegetables have softened, about 5 minutes. Drain fat from pan and set meat mixture aside.

3. In large soup pot or Dutch oven, heat beef stock over medium-high heat until boiling.

4. Add carrots and celery and cook until almost tender, about 5 minutes.

5. Add tomatoes, broccoli, parsley, seasonings and reserved meat mixture.

6. Mix well. Simmer over low heat 10 minutes until all vegetables are tender.

7. Taste and adjust seasonings.

41.   Low-carb Chicken Soup

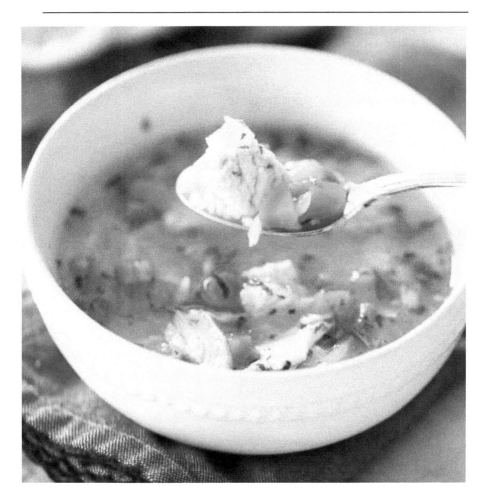

Ingredients:

- 2 leeks -- washed and sliced to 1" slices
- 3 turnips -- peeled, cut in chunks
- 1 bell pepper -- cut in 1" pieces
- 5 celery stalks -- cut in 1" pieces
- 4 chicken breast -- cut in bitesize pieces

- 32 ounces chicken broth -- I used a box variety2 cups water
- 1 clove garlic
- 1/4 teaspoon red pepper flakes
- 1 teaspoon salt
- fresh ground pepper to taste
- 1/2 teaspoon goya adobo seasoning
- 1/4 teaspoon thyme

Directions:

In large pot combine all ingredients and cook on low heat till turnips are tender.

Serves 6 to 8 hearty bowls.

42.   Quick Sausage Soup

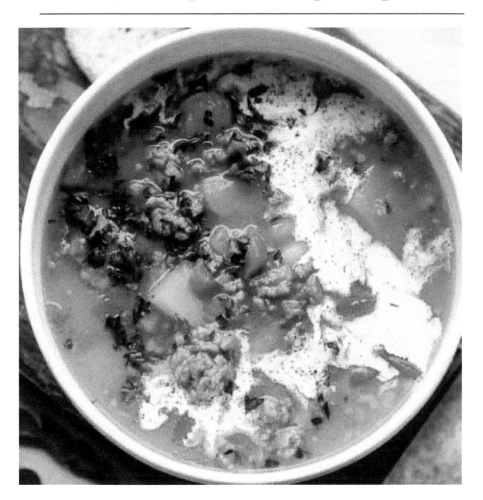

Ingredients:

- 1 pound ground pork sausage
- 3 tablespoons butter
- 1 1/2 tablespoons garlic -- crushed
- 1 1/2 tablespoons minced onion1 can beef broth
- 1 cup heavy cream

- 1 can green beans -- drained
- 1 cup carrots -- cooked
- pepper to taste

Directions:

1. Brown ground pork sausage in skillet.
2. In saucepan, melt butter.
3. Add garlic and onions and brown in melted butter.
4. Add sausage and remaining ingredients.
5. Heat thoroughly.

43.   Vegetable Soup

Ingredients:

- leftover roast beef - shredded or cut up - add au jus and water
- 1/2 medium onion -- cut up
- 1/2 green pepper -- cut up
- 4 medium mushrooms -- cut up
- 1 clove garlic -- chopped fine
- 1/2 head cauliflower -- cut in florets
- 1/2 cup celery -- finely chopped
- salt and pepper -- to taste
- cajun seasoning -- to taste

Directions:

Simmer all ingredients in soup pot for several hours. Eat Hardy!!!

44. Hearty Beef Stew

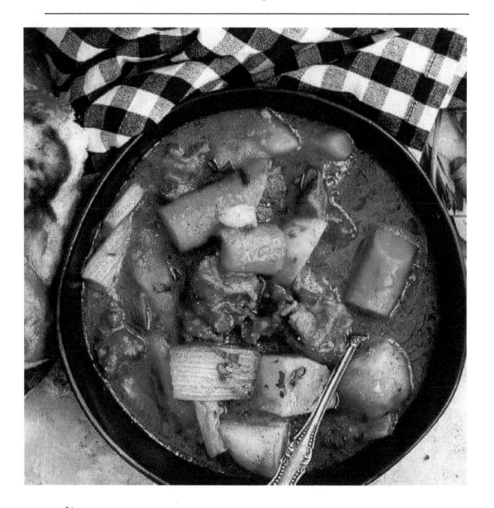

Ingredients:

- 1 1/2 pounds beef stew meat
- 14 1/2 ounces stewed tomatoes (1 can)
- 14 1/2 ounces beef broth (1 can)
- 1 cube beef bouillon
- 1/2 teaspoon onion powder

- 1/4 teaspoon garlic powder1 teaspoon salt
- 1/4 teaspoon pepper
- 1/4 teaspoon thyme
- 1 large rutabaga -- (or two small turnips)
- 2 medium zucchini

Directions:

1. Brown stew beef in olive oil on all sides in medium high pot. Add tomatoes, broth, spices and water to cover beef.
2. Turn heat down and simmer for about 1 and 1/2 hours.
3. Add cubed (about 1 inch) rutabagas and simmer for 30 minutes.
4. Add diced zucchini and simmer for 30 more minutes.
5. Add more liquid if necessary (to cover the veggies).
6. Taste for seasonings.

Lightning Source UK Ltd.
Milton Keynes UK
UKHW020740150621
385538UK00001B/25